This book has been sponsored by Ethicon Endo-Surgery (Europe) GmbH and Johnson & Johnson MEDICAL GmbH, Norderstedt, Germany. The authors are responsible for the content of the publication. Information provided in this book is offered in good faith as an educational tool for health care professionals. The information has been thoroughly reviewed and is believed to be useful and accurate at the time of its publication, but is offered without warranty of any kind. The authors and the sponsors shall not be responsible for any loss or damage arising from its use.

Operation Primer

THYROIDECTOMY
with Harmonic Focus®

Editors

Marc Immenroth
Thorsten Berg
Jürgen Brenner

Authors

Paolo Miccoli
Piero Berti
Thierry Defechereux

assisted by

Ann-Katrin Güler
Birgit Wahl
Christofer Coenen

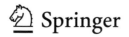 Springer

Authors

Paolo Miccoli, M.D.
Head of the Surgical Department, University of Pisa,
Via Roma 67, 56100, Pisa, Italy

Piero Berti, M.D.
Department of Surgery, University of Pisa,
Via Roma 67, 56100, Pisa, Italy

Thierry Defechereux, M.D., PhD
Assistant Professor in the Department of Endocrine, Breast & Transplant Surgery,
University Hospital CHU, Sart-Tilman B35, 4000 Liège, Belgium

Editors

Marc Immenroth, PhD
European Clinical Studies Manager, Ethicon Endo-Surgery (Europe) GmbH,
Hummelsbütteler Steindamm 71, 22851 Norderstedt, Germany

Thorsten Berg, M.D.
Director Outcomes Research, Johnson & Johnson Medical Pty Ltd,
1–5 Khartoum Road, North Ryde, NSW 2113, Australia

Jürgen Brenner, M.D.
Director European Surgical Institute, a division of Johnson & Johnson MEDICAL GmbH,
Hummelsbütteler Steindamm 71, 22851 Norderstedt, Germany

ISBN 978-3-540-85163-9 Thyroidectomy with Harmonic Focus®

Bibliografische Information der Deutschen Bibliothek
The Deutsche Bibliothek lists this publication in Deutsche Nationalbibliographie;
detailed bibliographic data are available in the internet at http://dnb.ddb.de.

First published in Germany in 2008 by Springer Medizin Verlag
springer.com

SPIN 12438457
Layout and typesetting: Dr. Carl GmbH, Stuttgart, Germany
Printing: Stürtz GmbH, Würzburg, Germany

18/5135/DK – 5 4 3 2 1 0

Editors' preface

The idea for the Operation Primer originated in a scientific study entitled "Mental Training in Surgical Education" that formed part of a collaborative project between the surgical department of the University of Cologne, the Institute of Sports and Sport Sciences of the University of Heidelberg and the European Surgical Institute (ESI) in Norderstedt.

The aim of the study was to evaluate the effect of mental training, which has been used successfully in top-class sports for decades, on surgical training. However, in order for mental training to be applied to surgery, it first had to undergo modification. In the course of this modification, the first Operation Primer was produced, the layout of which was largely adopted for the final version presented here.

Over several years the design of the Operation Primer was optimized and applied to other operations. At the same time, a team of authors was found who could transform the concept into a series of practical surgical primers. For this Operation Primer our first and very special thanks go to the authors Paolo Miccoli, Piero Berti and Thierry Defechereux, without whom it would not have been possible even to begin to think of converting our ideas into reality.

The text of the Operation Primer is fully comprehendible only when used in conjunction with the accompanying photographs. We would like to thank Lennart Wiman, who made and edited the pictures featured in the Operation Primer.

Reality often requires an abstraction in order to make certain situations clearer. This was the reason for including line drawings throughout the Operation Primer. These diagrams were produced by Thomas Heller, whom we gratefully acknowledge.

Our concept of practical surgical primers will become a reality through Dr. Carl GmbH and Springer Medizin Verlag Heidelberg.

The Operation Primers will be produced with the aim of describing the various operations in the simplest possible manner, but without over-simplifying. Although most time has been spent on the establishment of the scientific basis behind the operations, the main focus has always been on the practical relevance of the Primers.

With this Operation Primer we hope we have met our own as well as the readers' highest expectations.

The Editors   October 2008

Authors' preface

Thyroid surgery has progressed incredibly during the past 10 years. The technical improvements made possible by a strong integration between industry and surgeons are probably the most important reason for this outstanding progress. An important contribution to the development of energy devices was made by a series of key opinion leaders who gave their suggestions, if not in terms of engineering, in terms of ergonomics and flexibility. The latest product of this fruitful cooperation is the new Harmonic® device called Harmonic FOCUS®, which, I am quite sure, will constitute a milestone in the field of energy technology.

Paolo Miccoli   October 2008

We have been using ultrasonic technology for the past 10 years, both in abdominal and neck surgery. The evolution of this class of devices has been astonishing.
The latest innovation characterized by a new design and significant technical improvements is Harmonic FOCUS®. This intuitive and highly ergonomic instrument is going to change surgeons' approach to the neck. Not only thyroid and parathyroid operations, but also lymphadenectomies will benefit greatly from this new-generation Harmonic® tool.
The scientific literature will soon reflect the feelings we had when we began to use Harmonic FOCUS®.

Piero Berti   October 2008

It has been a long road since the Cooper project was initiated; the result is now available as the "Harmonic FOCUS®" device. Harmonic FOCUS® is a great accomplishment for Ethicon Endo-Surgery, and it is a wonderful opportunity for Head and Neck and Endocrine Surgeons to have at their disposal a device devoted and designed for the special requirements of their practice. The result of 3 years of research, including listening to "the voice of the customer", is a device so efficient and so comfortable that all initial users immediately abandon their previous instrument of choice. Ergonomics and the possibility for delicate dissection are no longer lacking. Combined with the safety and efficiency of the ultrasonic energy, these are the keys to the success of Harmonic FOCUS®. The device has changed the way we can perform a safe thyroidectomy in many ways. I am an enthusiastic user of it.

Thierry Defechereux   October 2008

Authors

Paolo Miccoli, M.D.

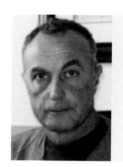

– Studied Medicine in Pisa, Italy
– Since 1986 Professor and Head of Department of Surgery at the
  University of Pisa, Italy

Founding member and memberships
– Former Councelor of the International Association of Endocrine Surgery and
  vice-president of Association Francophone de Chirurgie Endocrinienne
– Since 1995 Honorary Member of the Academie de Chirurgie of Paris
– Founder and former President of the European Society of Endocrine Surgeons
  and President of the Italian Society of Head and Neck Surgery
– Former President of the Italian Society of Endolaparoscopic Surgery and present
  President of the Club of Italian Endocrine Surgery

Experience
He performs around 500 thyroid operations per year. Around 100 surgeons visit his
operating theatre every year.
He conceived the first operation in video-assisted endoscopic surgery without gas
insufflations to remove the parathyroid's adenomas and thyroid glands.

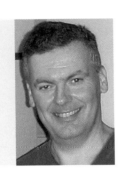

Piero Berti, M.D.

– Studied Medicine in Pisa, Italy
– 1986–1988 Intern in the Division of General Surgery at the University of Pisa, Italy
– 1988 Doctorate in Medicine at the University of Pisa, Italy
– Since 1997 contribution to the improvement of minimally invasive surgery together with Prof. P. Miccoli, developing a minimally invasive, video-assisted technique for thyroidectomy and parathyroidectomy
– Since 2003 Associate Professor at the University of Pisa, Italy

Teaching activities
– First Operator in several videolaparoscopic and video-assisted operations in the context of workshops, post-graduate courses and live and telesurgery sessions at the University of Pisa and around the world
– Expert in several workshops and courses for general practitioners and surgeons
– Teacher with a temporary appointment at the Specialization Schools of General Surgery, Vascular Surgery, Endocrinology, Anaesthesia of the University of Pisa

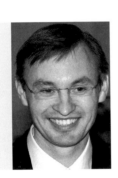

Thierry Defechereux, M.D., PhD

– Studied Medicine in Liège, Belgium
– 1996 Diploma in Surgery, Fellowship in Endocrine surgery in Marseilles, France
– 2000 Doctor (PhD) in Medical Science
– Since 2001 Assistant Professor in the Department of Endocrine, Breast & Transplant Surgery at the University Hospital CHU in Liège, Belgium
– 2007 European Board of Surgery: Qualification in European Endocrine Surgery

Memberships
– Member of the Belgian Royal Society of Surgery (SRBC)
– Executive committee of the French-speaking Association of Endocrine Surgery (AFCE)
– Member of International Association of Endocrine Surgery (IAES)
– Member of International Society of Surgery (ISS/SIC)
– Corresponding Member of American Association of Endocrine Surgery (AAES)
– Corresponding member of British Association of Endocrine Surgery (BAES)
– Editorial Board of Langenbeck's Archives of Surgery
– Executive committee of the European Society of Endocrine Surgeons (ESES)

Editors

Marc Immenroth, PhD

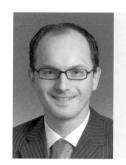

- Studied Psychology (Diploma) and Sports Science (Master) in Heidelberg, Germany
- 1999–2006 Sport Psychologist (including consultant to many German top athletes during their preparation for the World Championships and Olympics) and Industrial Psychologist (including consultant to Lufthansa Inc.)
- 2000 Research Scientist at the University of Greifswald, Germany (Policlinic for Restorative Dentistry and Periodontology)
- 2001–2004 Research Scientist at the University of Heidelberg, Germany (Institute of Sports and Sports Science)
- 2002 Doctorate in Psychology at the University of Heidelberg, Germany
- 2005–2006 Assistant Lecturer at the University of Giessen, Germany (Institute of Sport)
- 2006 –2008 Assistant Professor at the University of Greifswald, Germany (Institute of Sport)
- Since 2006 European Clinical Studies Manager at Ethicon Endo-Surgery Europe in Norderstedt, Germany

Focus of Research and Work
- Mental Training in Sport, Surgery and Aviation
- Virtual Reality in Surgical Education
- Coping with Emotion and Stress

Author of many scientific articles and textbooks in psychology, sports science and medicine

Thorsten Berg, M.D.

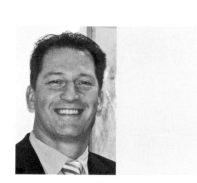

- Studied Medicine in Heidelberg, Germany
- 1996 Intern at the University Hospital, Durban, South Africa
- 1997 Intern at the Surgical Department of the General Hospital, Ludwigshafen, Germany
- 2003 Qualified as General Surgeon
- 2003 Director of Education of European Surgical Institute in Norderstedt, Germany
- 2005 Director of Clinical Development at Ethicon Endo-Surgery Europe in Norderstedt, Germany
- 2006 Senior Manager Health Outcome at Ethicon Endo-Surgery Europe in Norderstedt, Germany
- 2007 Doctorate in Medicine at the University of Heidelberg, Germany
- Since 2008 Director Outcomes Research at Johnson & Johnson Medical in Sydney, Australia

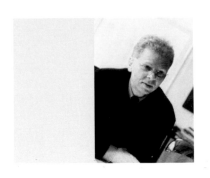

Jürgen Brenner, M.D.

- Studied Medicine in Hamburg, Germany
- 1972 Medical Doctor at University of Hamburg, Germany
- 1972 Institute for Neuroanatomy, University of Hamburg, Germany
- 1974 Senior Resident at the Department of Surgery of the General Hospital Hamburg-Wandsbek, Germany
- 1981 Medical Director of Department for Colorectal and Trauma Surgery at St. Adolf Stift Hospital in Reinbek, Germany
- 1987 Director for Surgical Research of Ethicon Inc. in Norderstedt, Germany
- 1989 Director of European Surgical Institute and Vice President Professional Education Europe of Ethicon Endo-Surgery Europe in Norderstedt, Germany
- 2004 Managing Director Ethicon Endo-Surgery Germany in Norderstedt, Germany
- Since 2008 Director of European Surgical Institute in Norderstedt, Germany

Assistants

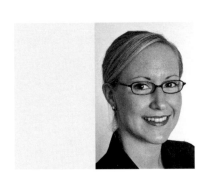

Ann-Katrin Güler

- Studied Medicine in Hamburg, Germany
- Since 2005 doctoral thesis 'Development and evaluation of standardized operation primer for education in minimal invasive surgery' at the University of Hamburg, Germany (Department of General, Thoracic and Visceral Surgery)
- Since 2007 member of the Market Access department at Ethicon Endo-Surgery Europe in Norderstedt, Germany

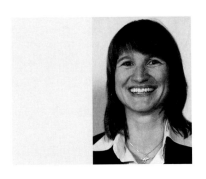

Birgit Wahl, M.D.

- Studied Medicine in Freiburg, Germany
- 2000–2003 Intern at different Surgical Departments, Germany
- 2003 Doctorate in Medicine at the University of Freiburg, Germany
- 2003–2006 Product Manager at Spitta Publishing House in Balingen, Germany
- Since 2006 Free Medical Writer at Dr. Carl GmbH in Stuttgart, Germany
- Since 2008 certified Medical Journalist, Deutsche Fachjournalisten-Schule in Berlin, Germany

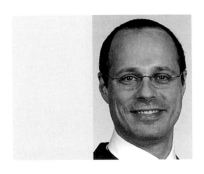

Christofer Coenen, M.D.

- Studied Medicine in Freiburg, Germany
- 1999 Doctorate in Medicine at the University of Freiburg, Germany
- 1999–2001 Intern at Department of Medicine of the General Hospital, Bruchsal, Germany
- 2001–2002 Postgraduate study "Medical Knowledge Management" at the University of Heidelberg, Germany
- Since 2002 Project Manager and Medical Writer at Dr. Carl GmbH in Stuttgart, Germany

Contents

IV Anatomical variations

Appendix

Introduction

From an educational point of view, the Operation Primer is somewhat plagiaristic. The layout – and this can be admitted freely – is largely taken over from commonly available cook books. In such books, the ingredients and cooking utensils required to prepare the recipe in question are normally listed first. The most important cooking procedures are then described briefly in the text. Photographs support the written explanations and show what the dish should look like when prepared. Sometimes diagrams and illustrations make individual cooking steps clearer.

Despite these obvious parallels, there is a crucial difference between cook books and the Operation Primer: in the Operation Primer, complicated and complex surgical techniques are described that are intended to help the surgeon and his team perform an operation safely and economically. Ultimately, it always comes down to the patient's welfare. The following must therefore be said early in this introduction:

- The use of the Operation Primer as an aid to operating requires that surgical techniques have first been completely mastered.

- Being alert to possible mistakes is categorically the most important principle when operating; avoiding mistakes is crucial.

As already mentioned in the Editors' preface, the concept of the Operation Primer originated in a scientific study with the title "Mental Training in Surgical Education" that formed part of a collaborative project between the surgical department of the University of Cologne (under Prof. Hans Troidl), the Institute of Sports and Sport Science of the University of Heidelberg and the European Surgical Institute (ESI) in Norderstedt. Laparoscopic cholecystectomy was the initial focus.

Mental training is derived from top-class sports. This is understood as the methodically repeated and conscious imagination of actions and movements without actually carrying them out at the same time (cf. Driskell, Copper & Moran, 1994; Ebers-pächer, 2001; Feltz & Landers, 1983; Immenroth, 2003). Scientific involvement with imagining movement has a long tradition in medical and psychological research. As early as 1852, Lotze described how imagining and perceiving movements can lead to a concurrent performance "with quiet movements …" (Lotze, 1852). This phenomenon later became known by the names "Ideomotion" and "Carpenter effect" (Carpenter, 1874).

In the collaborative project, mental training was modified in such a way that it could be employed in the training and further education of young surgeons. In mental training in surgery, surgeons imagine the operation from the inner perspective without performing any actual movements, i.e. they go through the operation step by step in their mind's eye. In the study that was conducted at the European Surgical Institute (ESI), the first Operation Primer was used as the basis for this imagination. In this primer, laparoscopic cholecystectomy was subdivided into individual, clearly depicted steps, the so-called nodal points.

The study evaluated the effect of the mental training on learning laparoscopic cholecystectomy compared with practical training and with a control group. The planning, conducting and evaluation of the study took 7 years (2000–2007), with over 100 surgeons participating.

The results corresponded exactly with the expectations: the mentally trained surgeons improved in a similar degree to those surgeons who received additional practical training on a pelvi trainer simulator (in some subscales even more). Moreover, there was greater improvement in these two groups compared with the control group, which did not receive any additional mental or practical training (cf. in detail, Immenroth, Bürger, Brenner, Nagelschmidt, Eberspächer & Troidl, 2007; Immenroth, Bürger, Brenner, Kemmler, Nagelschmidt, Eberspächer & Troidl, 2005; Immenroth, Eberspächer, Nagelschmidt, Troidl, Bürger, Brenner, Berg, Müller & Kemmler, 2005).

Furthermore, the study included a questionnaire to determine the extent to which the mentally trained surgeons accepted mental training as a teaching method in surgery. Mental training was assessed as very positive by all 34 mentally trained surgeons. The Operation Primer received particular acclaim in the evaluation (cf. in detail, Immenroth et al., 2007):

- 28 surgeons wished to use similar self-made Operation Primers in their daily work.

- 29 surgeons attributed the success of the mental training at least in part to the Operation Primer.

- 30 surgeons wanted to have these Operation Primers as a fixed component of the course at the European Surgical Institute (ESI).

This positive response to the study was the starting point for the production of the present series of Operation Primers.

Prior to publication, the Operation Primer was developed by methodical and didactical means and then adapted to the readers' needs and wishes. This was carried out following a survey of 93 surgeons (interns, resident doctors, assistant medical directors and medical directors) who participated in surgical courses at the European Surgical Institute (ESI). They evaluated in detail the structure and components by means of a questionnaire.

The results of this survey gave important findings on how to optimize the Operation Primer. The sense and representation of the nodal points, the comprehensibility and detail of the text, and the photographs of the operation were highly valued especially by young surgeons (Güler, Immenroth, Berg, Bürger & Gawad, 2006). The comprehensive research undertaken with this Operation Primer series will ensure its overall value to the reader.

Structure and handling of the Operation Primer

In the present series of Operation Primers, an attempt has been made to standardize the described operations as much as possible. This is achieved on the one hand by applying the same structure to all operational techniques described. On the other hand, operative sequences that are performed identically in all operations are always explained by using the same blocks of text. By following a general structure for the description of all operations and by using identical text blocks, it was intended to aid recognition of recurring patterns and their translation into action even for different operations.

The Operation Primer is divided into four chapters, each identified by Roman numerals and different register colors on the margin. The contents of the individual chapters will now be explained.

In **Preparations for the operation,** the instruments for the operation are listed. This is followed by a detailed description of the positioning and shaving of the patient, attaching the neutral electrode, setting the equipment, skin disinfection and sterile draping of the patient. The operative preparation is concluded with a detailed description and picture of how the operating team is to be positioned for the operation in question.

The core of the Operation Primer is the chapter **Nodal points.** This is where the actual sequence of the operation is described in detail. However, prior to this detailed explanation, the term nodal point will be covered briefly. In the Editors' preface and the introduction, mental training was mentioned as a form of training used successfully in top-class sports for decades, and this is where the term originates. In sports as in surgery, a nodal point is understood as one of those structural components of movement that are absolutely essential for performing the movement optimally. Nodal points have to be passed through in succession and are characterized by a reduction in the degrees of freedom of action. In mental training they act as orientation points for methodically repeated and conscious imagination of the athletic movement or operation (cf. in detail Immenroth, Eberspächer & Hermann, 2008).

For every operation in the Operation Primer series, these nodal points were extracted in a prolonged process by the authors in collaboration with the editors. The nodal points represent the basic structural framework of an operation. Because of their particular relevance and for better orientation, all of the nodal points in the Operation Primer are shown on the left on each double page as a flow chart. The current nodal point is highlighted graphically. An anatomical graphic of the operative situs and the instruments required for this nodal point are listed in a box on the right beside the flow chart.

Below the instrument box, instructions regarding the nodal point are given as briefly as possible. Based on the ideas of Miller (1956), according to whom people can best store 7 ± 2 information units ("Magical number 7"), not more than seven single instructions per nodal point are listed, if possible. With regard to the instructions, it should be noted that the change of instruments between the individual nodal points is not described explicitly as a rule; rather, this is apparent through different instruments in the instrument box.

I	Preparations for the operation
II	Nodal points
III	Management of difficult situations, complications and mistakes
VI	Anatomical variations
	Appendix

**Nodal point =
term from top-class sports**

**Nodal points:
1) absolutely essential
2) successive order
3) no degrees of freedom**

**Flow chart of the sequence
of nodal points on each
double page**

**Continuous illustration
of the operative situs**

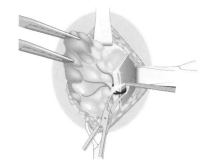

**Maximum of 7 ± 2 instructions
per nodal point**

Danger warnings are pointed out in red!

Where necessary, particular moments of danger are pointed out in red.

The described operation sequence is only one way of performing the operation safely and economically, namely the way preferred by the authors. Undoubtedly, a number of other equally valid operation sequences exist. As far as possible, notes on alternative methods are given in small blue print at the end of each nodal point.

Alternatives: In small blue print at the end of the nodal point.

In the third chapter, the **Management of difficult situations, complications and mistakes** is described in detail. In general, details on adhesions, bleeding, injuries to organs, etc. are given first.

Illustration of the most important anatomical variations

The following chapter goes into relevant **Anatomical variations** which can occur in the described operation sequence and may require a different approach. In order to provide a clear description, only the most important anatomical variations are mentioned.

Example of an operation note in the appendix

In order to give the Operation Primer even more practical relevance, an example of an operation note is reproduced in the **Appendix.** Besides the operation note, the appendix also contains the bibliographical references and list of key words.

(→ p. 51, III-2) = reference to the 2nd section of chapter III

In order to avoid repetition, reference is made throughout the text to relevant chapters of the Operation Primer if necessary. To do this, the Roman numeral of the chapter and the number of the corresponding section are shown in parentheses. Referral is made most often to the third chapter where the management of difficult situations, complications and mistakes is described. These references are set off in red letters.

All sources in the literature are listed in the bibliography

Additionally, it must be pointed out that for better readability of the Operation Primer no bibliographical references at all are given in the text. However, in order to give an overview of the basic and more extensive sources, the entire literature is listed in the bibliography.

The Harmonic® system

Equipment

The Harmonic® system enables hemostatic cutting and/or coagulation of soft tissue utilizing ultrasonic energy.

The system consists of an ultrasonic generator, a footswitch, optional a hand-switching adapter, a hand piece and a variety of open and minimally invasive instruments.

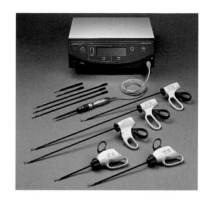

The Harmonic FOCUS® shears are indicated for soft-tissue incisions when bleeding control and minimal thermal injury are desired. They allow cutting and coagulation of vessels up to and including 5 mm in diameter.

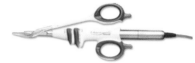

Working principles

Electrical energy from the generator is converted into ultrasonic vibration in a piezoelectric ceramic system. An acoustic mount coupled to the housing of the hand piece transfers the energy to the blade system.

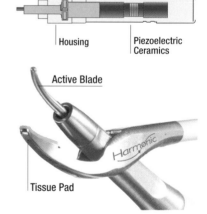

Mount   Transducer

Housing   Piezoelectric Ceramics

The active blade of the instrument vibrates axially 55.500 times per second (Hz). The amplitude of the vibration can be varied between 25 and 100 μm in five levels at the generator (→ p. 27).

Active Blade

Tissue Pad

Notes for use

Harmonic® yields four tissue effects, which can be applied solely or in synergistic combination to the tissue.

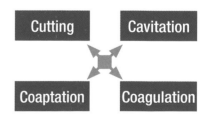

Cutting   Cavitation

Coaptation   Coagulation

Cutting

Cutting with Harmonic® is done primarily by the surgeon's hand movements but also by the mechanical ultrasound wave moving the active blade of the instrument.

To achieve the cutting effect it is necessary to prestretch the tissue close to its elastic limit, due to the so-called rubber-band phenomenon: if the scalpel were applied to an unstretched rubber band, the rubber band would retreat, owing to its elasticity, but if it is stretched, a light touch is enough to cut it through.

Cutting speed depends on generator level, tissue condition and blade sharpness.

Cavitation

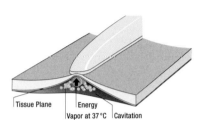

Tissue Plane | Energy
Vapor at 37 °C | Cavitation

The vibrating tip of the active blade produces exhaustive transient pressure changes in the tissue, which cause intercellular and intracellular water to vaporize at body temperature (= cavitation).

The cavitational effect causes water to expand between tissue planes and facilitates exact anatomical preparation.

During cavitation, a fine mist of water is released. The intensity of the resulting mist depends mainly on tissue condition and tissue water content.

Cavitation is a side effect which becomes apparent whenever ultrasound energy is used and runs coincidentally with cutting, coaptation and coagulation.

Coaptation

The vibration of the active blade causes defragmentation and collapse of proteins by breaking tertiary hydrogen bonds below 63 °C.

When coaptation is achieved and pressure is applied to vessel walls, it is possible to seal and divide the vessel with sufficient hemostasis.

Coagulation

Application of energy for a longer period (i.e. a few seconds), in combination with pressure, allows sufficient hemostasis.

Vibrating proteins produce secondary heat that leads to protein denaturation (at > 63 °C) and causes coagulation.

The balance between cutting and coagulation can be controlled by

• changing the generator power level,

• varying traction and tension,

• varying grip pressure,

• selecting a special blade or blade side.

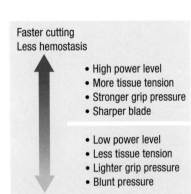

Faster cutting
Less hemostasis

• High power level
• More tissue tension
• Stronger grip pressure
• Sharper blade

• Low power level
• Less tissue tension
• Lighter grip pressure
• Blunt pressure

Slower cutting
More hemostasis

- No electricity passing through patient or surgeon
- Precise cutting and coagulation
- Minimal thermal tissue damage
- Minimal lateral spread of energy
- Better visualization of the operating field (reduces smoke, mist or vapor)
- Few instrument changes necessary
- Shorter operating time and less pain (compared with electrocautery)

Precise knowledge and understanding of the technical basis and characteristics of Harmonic® is a fundamental requirement for the successful use of Harmonic®!

The learning phase can be shortened by attending appropriate theoretical and practical courses!

Preparations for the operation

Make sure that the following preoperative requirements for thyroidectomy with Harmonic FOCUS® shears have been met:

• The indication for the operation is correct.

• The patient has given detailed written consent.

• A blood test has been performed to ascertain the euthyroidism and exclude a thyroiditis.

• Ultrasonography of the thyroid gland has been done.

• Scintigraphy of the thyroid gland has been done.

• A fine-needle aspiration biopsy has been performed, if a suspicious nodule has been shown by ultrasonography.

• An X-ray examination of the trachea and the thorax and a barium study of the esophagus have been performed, if any suspicion of an intrathoracic goiter or a tracheal deviation is present.

• A laryngoscopic examination to evaluate the motility of the vocal cords has been performed by an otorhinolaryngologist.

• The location of the tentative skin incision has been marked.

• Thrombosis prophylaxis (low-molecular-weight heparin), if mandatory, has been given.

Instruments

• 2 Langenbeck retractors
• Scalpel blade 15
• 3 atraumatic forceps
• 2 surgical forceps
• Metzenbaum scissors
• Mayo scissors
• Scissors
• 2 Needle holders
• 4 straight clamps
• 6 Mosquito hemostats
• 2 Péan clamps
• 10 curved clamps
• 3 hemostatic forceps
• 3 Backhaus clamps
• Drain needle
• Nurse scissors
• Compresses
• Swabs

- Sutures:
  - Absorbable sutures for the retaining suture
  - Absorbable sutures for ligatures, if necessary
  - Absorbable sutures for sewing the strap muscles, if necessary
  - Absorbable sutures for dividing the isthmus, if necessary
  - Midline: 2–0 absorbable
  - Platysma: 3–0 absorbable
  - Skin: 5–0 absorbable, monofilament
- HF (high-frequency) cautery electrode handle and forceps
- Suction device
- Clip applier with clips, if necessary
- 2 Redon's suction drainages, if necessary
- Surgicell fibrillar, if necessary
- Dressings

- Harmonic FOCUS® shears with blue hand piece (Ethicon Endo-Surgery)

Before using Harmonic FOCUS® shears read the instructions for use and become familiar with the instrument!

Be aware that the Harmonic FOCUS® shears instrument may heat up during use. Therefore, avoid unintended contact with tissue, drapes, surgical gowns, or other unintended sites at all times!

- Neuromonitoring device (e.g. Neurosign 100®, courtesy of inomed Medizintechnik GmbH)

Neuromonitoring is recommended to avoid damage of neural structures (→ p. 51, III-2; p. 52, III-3)!

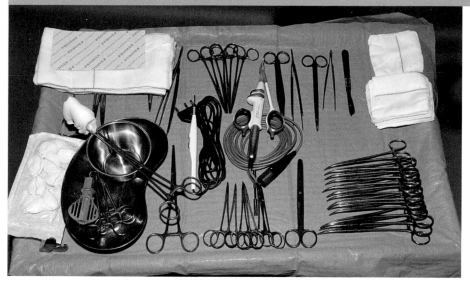

Positioning of the patient

- Put the patient in supine position.

- Place a pad under the shoulders to obtain a moderate hyperextension of the neck.

- Position a sponge doughnut under the patient's head.

- Then elevate the head of the table to a 30° position.

- Place the right arm alongside the body and the left arm at an angle no greater than 70° to the long axis of the body in order to avoid injuries to the axillary nerve.

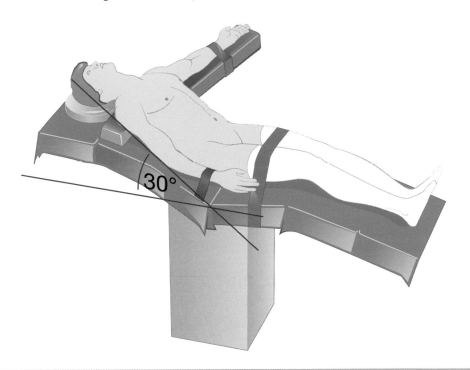

Shaving

- Shave the area of the patient's upper thorax up to the chin, if necessary.

- If monopolar current is used, shave the adhesion side for the neutral electrode (as close as possible to the operating field, e.g. on the lateral abdomen).

Neutral electrode

- Before placing the neutral electrode, ensure that the skin at this site and all skin areas in contact with the table are absolutely dry.

- Then stick the entire surface of the electrode carefully above the greatest possible muscle mass. The conducting cable must be at the greatest possible distance from the operating field.

When using monopolar current, always guard against burns on moist areas of the skin due to current!

- The Harmonic FOCUS® shears instrument is designed exclusively for use with the Harmonic® Generator 300.

Before using the Harmonic® Generator 300 read the instructions for use and the service manual!

- Set the Harmonic® Generator 300 and the generator of HF (high-frequency) cautery to an appropriate power level for the intended use.

- Position the foot pedal.

- Attach the suction device.

- Disinfect the skin of the chin, the ventral and lateral collar, the ventrolateral shoulder girdle and the upper thorax. Pay particular attention to careful disinfection of all skin folds.

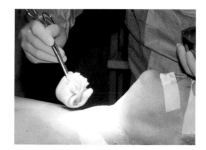

- Drape the operating field with adhesive sterile drapes so that it is limited cranially at the level of the chin, caudally just below the sternal notch, and laterally by the posterior margin of the sternocleidomastoid muscles.

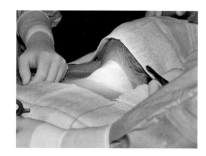

Positioning of the operating team

Supine position with moderate neck hyperextension

• The surgeon stands to the right at the level of the patient's shoulder.

• The first assistant stands to the left at the level of the patient's shoulder.

• The second assistant stands at the end of the table behind the patient's head.

• The instrument nurse stands to the right at the level of the patient's abdomen.

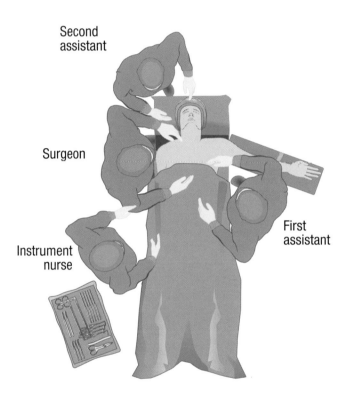

Nodal points

1 Incising the skin and the superficial cervical fascia

2 Exposing the thyroid

3 Preparing the thyroid and dividing the middle thyroid vein

4 Exposing the superior pole and dividing the superior thyroid vessels

5 Identifying the parathyroid glands

6 Identifying the recurrent laryngeal nerve and dividing the inferior thyroid artery

7 Dissecting the inferior pole and dividing the inferior thyroid vein

8 Mobilizing the thyroid lobe

9 Finishing the operation

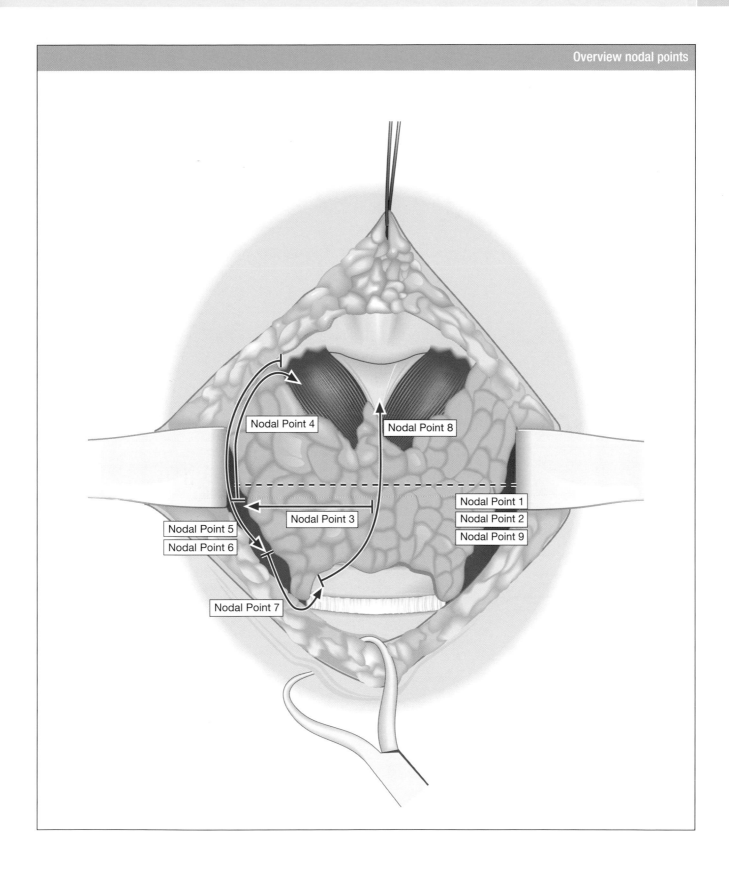

Nodal point 1

Incising the skin and the superficial cervical fascia

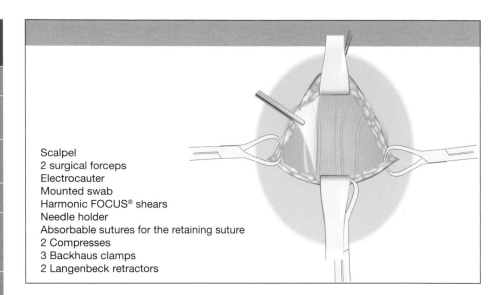

Scalpel
2 surgical forceps
Electrocauter
Mounted swab
Harmonic FOCUS® shears
Needle holder
Absorbable sutures for the retaining suture
2 Compresses
3 Backhaus clamps
2 Langenbeck retractors

Perform with a scalpel a horizontal, curvilinear skin incision approximately 2 cm above the sternal notch and about 6–8 cm in length in between the two sternocleidomastoid muscles in a skin fold (Kocher collar incision). The exact length of the incision depends on the size of the thyroid and on cosmetic concerns.

> Perform the skin incision in an optimal length and at the preferred position in order to avoid keloid formation and therefore an unsatisfactory cosmetic outcome!

Incise the subcutaneous fat and the platysma horizontally with an electrocauter or a scalpel.

Dissect the subcutaneous fat and the platysma from the underlying cervical fascia and the anterior jugular veins partly with a mounted swab or finger (blunt dissection), partly with Harmonic FOCUS® shears (sharp dissection). Continue dissecting above the cervical fascia in cranial direction up to the thyroid cartilage and also in caudal direction until the sternal notch.

Position a retaining suture at the cranial margin of the incision. Then place two compresses around the wound and fix them at the caudal and lateral margins of the incision with three Backhaus clamps. Insert two Langenbeck retractors at the cranial and caudal margin of the incision to keep it open.

Incise the superficial cervical fascia horizontally with Harmonic FOCUS® shears.

Dissect and seal the superficial collar veins with Harmonic FOCUS® shears. Take care to identify and preserve the anterior jugular veins.

> Make sure not to injure the anterior jugular veins (→ p. 51, III-1)!

> Alternative: Tie up the superficial collar veins using ligatures.

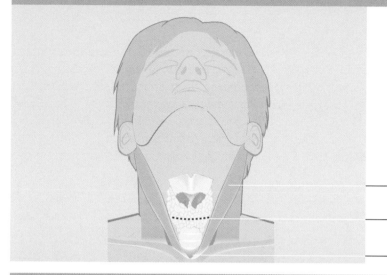

Sternocleidomastoid muscle

Kocher collar incision

Sternal notch

Incising the subcutaneous fat and the platysma

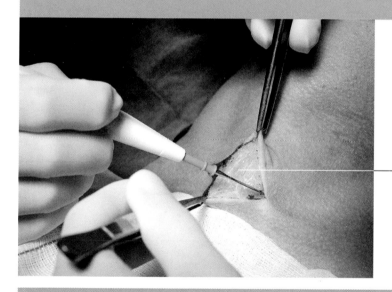

Subcutaneous fat and platysma

Identifying the superficial cervical fascia

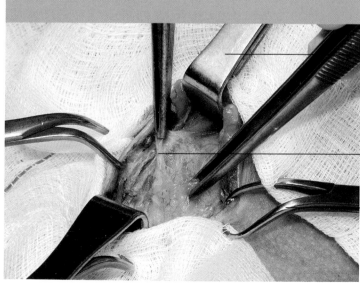

Langenbeck retractor

Superficial cervical fascia

Backhaus clamp

Nodal point 2 | **Exposing the thyroid**

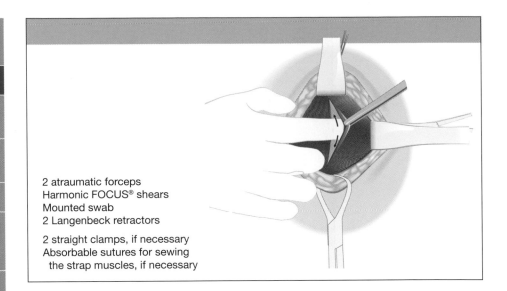

2 atraumatic forceps
Harmonic FOCUS® shears
Mounted swab
2 Langenbeck retractors

2 straight clamps, if necessary
Absorbable sutures for sewing
  the strap muscles, if necessary

Reposition the caudal Langenbeck retractor to the right lateral side of the incision.

Open the medial cervical fascia longitudinally over 3–4 cm in the midline between the strap muscles (cervical linca alba) with Harmonic FOCUS® shears. Coagulate small crossing vessels with Harmonic FOCUS® shears.

Identify the connective tissue layer (spatium chirurgicum De Quervain) between the strap muscles and the thyroid capsule.

Move the right lateral Langenbeck retractor to the left lateral side of the incision.

Then separate the strap muscles from the underlying thyroid capsule in this layer on both sides, partly bluntly with a mounted swab or finger, partly sharply with Harmonic FOCUS® shears. Take care not to injure the thyroid capsule and to perform accurate hemostasis.

> Separate the strap muscles from the thyroid capsule in the right connective tissue layer in order to avoid injuries of the thyroid capsule and to achieve sufficient hemostasis (→ p. 51, III-1)!

In case of a large struma, divide the strap muscles transversely in between two straight clamps with Harmonic FOCUS® shears. To avoid bleeding sew the cut ends of the muscles if necessary.

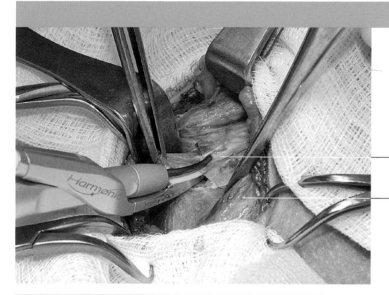

Medial cervical fascia

Strap muscle

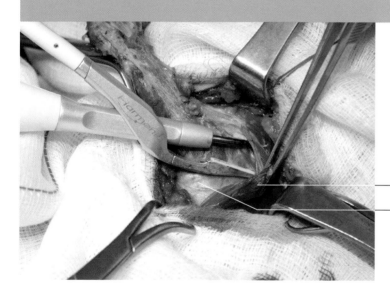

Strap muscle

Thyroid

Nodal point 3 | **Preparing the thyroid and dividing the middle thyroid vein**

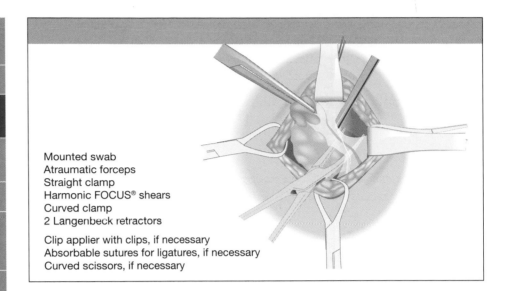

Mounted swab
Atraumatic forceps
Straight clamp
Harmonic FOCUS® shears
Curved clamp
2 Langenbeck retractors

Clip applier with clips, if necessary
Absorbable sutures for ligatures, if necessary
Curved scissors, if necessary

Prepare and resect first one, then the contralateral thyroid lobe, using the same technique for both sides, described as follows:

Prepare the forefront of the thyroid lobe towards the lateral side of the gland by shoving away the connective tissue between the thyroid capsule and the soft parts of the collar with a mounted swab or finger.

Then carefully draw the thyroid lobe to the contralateral side with a straight clamp in order to open the lateral space. Be careful not to disrupt the middle thyroid vein.

> Be careful not to disrupt the middle thyroid vein while dissecting the lateral part of the thyroid gland (→ p. 51, III-1)!

Open the superficial fascia between the thyroid gland and the carotid sheath with Harmonic FOCUS® shears carefully. Make sure not to damage the pericarotid plexus running next to the carotid sheath.

> Pay attention to the pericarotid plexus to avoid any injuries (→ p. 52, III-4)!

Isolate the middle thyroid vein from the surrounding tissue with a curved clamp and seal it with Harmonic FOCUS® shears.

> In case of a large diameter (> 5 mm) of the middle thyroid vein, it is mandatory to clip or ligate the vein with absorbable suture and cut it with curved scissors (→ p. 51, III-1)!

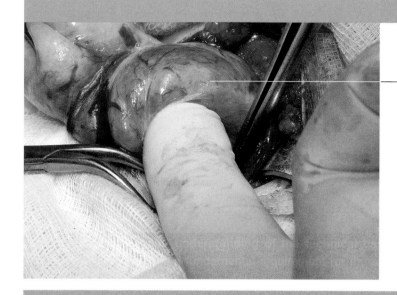

Thyroid lobe

Isolating the middle thyroid vein

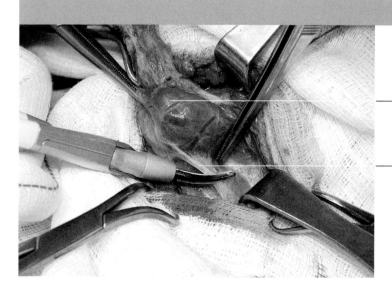

Thyroid lobe

Middle thyroid vein

Curved clamp

Sealing the middle thyroid vein

Thyroid lobe

Middle thyroid vein

Nodal point 4 — Exposing the superior pole and dividing the superior thyroid vessels

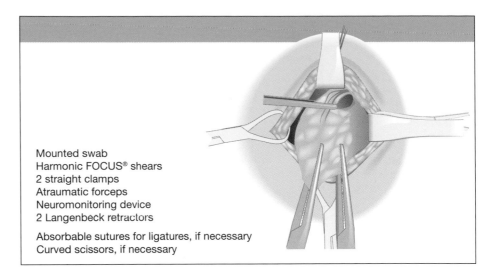

Mounted swab
Harmonic FOCUS® shears
2 straight clamps
Atraumatic forceps
Neuromonitoring device
2 Langenbeck retractors

Absorbable sutures for ligatures, if necessary
Curved scissors, if necessary

Dissect the thyroid gland laterally towards the superior pole of the lobe in the connective tissue layer partly bluntly with a mounted swab, partly sharply with Harmonic FOCUS® shears.

Retract the thyroid lobe caudally with two straight clamps and carefully prepare the superior pole close to the thyroid capsule. As the external branch of the superior laryngeal nerve runs in the adventitial tissue close to the superior thyroid artery and the larynx, it is important to identify the nerve prior to any division by using neuro-monitoring.

> Always make sure to identify the external branch of the superior laryngeal nerve before making any division (→ p. 52, III-3)!

After exposing the superior pole, open a window medially between the cricothyroid muscle of the larynx and the medial border of the superior pole with Harmonic FOCUS® shears.

Look for a pyramidal lobe (remnant of the thyroglossal duct). Mobilize and remove an existing pyramidal lobe as completely as possible with Harmonic FOCUS® shears.

> Remove an existing pyramidal lobe as completely as possible in order to avoid recurrences of the struma in the pyramidal lobe!

Seal and divide the distal branches of the superior thyroid vessels close to the thyroid capsule step by step with Harmonic FOCUS® shears. Keep the external branch of the superior laryngeal nerve in mind, which may run close to the vessels.

> If the diameter of the superior thyroid vessels is too large (> 5 mm), it is mandatory to ligate them selectively and close to the thyroid capsule with absorbable suture and to divide the vessels with curved scissors (→ p. 51, III-1)!

While going deeper into the tissue make sure not to damage the superior parathyroid gland and maintain some distance to the pericarotid plexus.

> Pay attention to the superior parathyroid gland and the pericarotid plexus to avoid any injuries (→ p. 52, III-4; p. 52, III-6)!

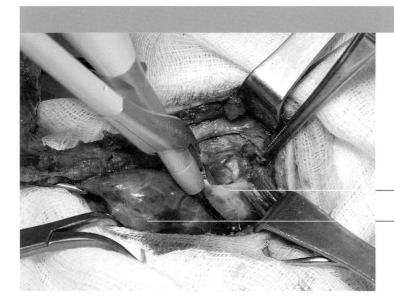

Superior thyroid vessels

Superior pole

Thyroid lobe

Dividing the superior thyroid vessels

Superior thyroid vessels

Thyroid lobe

Nodal point 5   Identifying the parathyroid glands

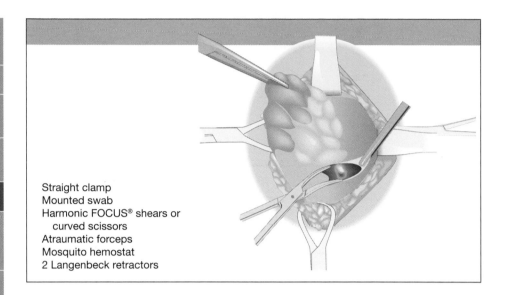

Straight clamp
Mounted swab
Harmonic FOCUS® shears or
   curved scissors
Atraumatic forceps
Mosquito hemostat
2 Langenbeck retractors

Draw the thyroid lobe gently to the opposite side with a straight clamp. Prepare the thyroid gland lateral and dorsal in caudal direction in the connective tissue layer partly bluntly with a mounted swab, partly sharply with Harmonic FOCUS® shears. During preparation, look for a possibly existing ectopic inferior parathyroid gland.

> Identify a possibly existing ectopic inferior parathyroid gland in order to avoid any injury to the gland (→ p. 52, III-6)!

Dissect and visualize the superior and inferior parathyroid gland at the back of the thyroid lobe with a Mosquito hemostat. Separate the parathyroid glands with their vascular pedicles from the posterior capsule of the thyroid carefully, with Harmonic FOCUS® shears or curved scissors.

> Take care to preserve the parathyroid glands with their native blood supply in order to avoid a postoperative hypoparathyroidism with hypocalcemia (→ p. 52, III-6)!

Thyroid lobe

Recurrent laryngeal nerve

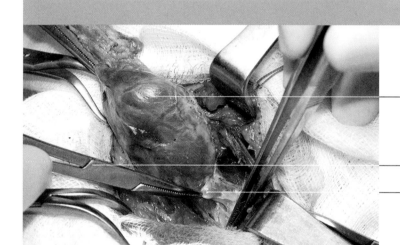

Thyroid lobe

Mosquito hemostat

Superior parathyroid gland

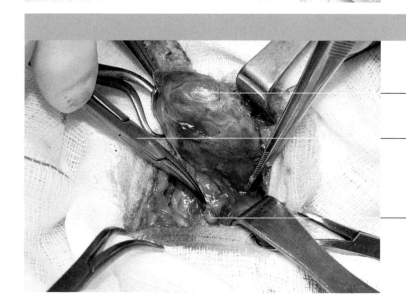

Thyroid lobe

Mosquito hemostat

Inferior parathyroid gland

Nodal point 6   **Identifying the recurrent laryngeal nerve and dividing the inferior thyroid arte**

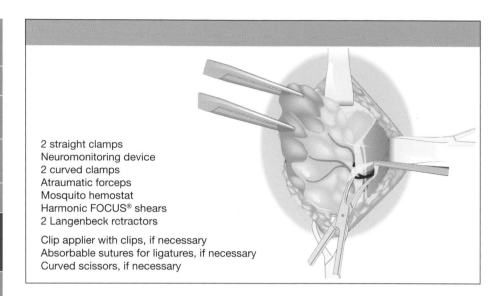

2 straight clamps
Neuromonitoring device
2 curved clamps
Atraumatic forceps
Mosquito hemostat
Harmonic FOCUS® shears
2 Langenbeck retractors

Clip applier with clips, if necessary
Absorbable sutures for ligatures, if necessary
Curved scissors, if necessary

Reposition the cranial Langenbeck retractor to the caudal margin of the incision.

Identify the recurrent laryngeal nerve, which runs at the back of the thyroid lobe in the thyrotracheal groove and crosses the inferior thyroid artery. Use neuromonitoring to identify the recurrent laryngeal nerve more quickly, or if the anatomical situation is complicated.

Dissect the inferior thyroid artery including its branches and the recurrent laryngeal nerve parallel to the anticipated course of the nerve very carefully with a curved clamp. Do not skeletonize the recurrent laryngeal nerve, and keep in mind that 5 mm is the minimal distance recommended for approaching it.

> Make sure to identify the recurrent laryngeal nerve clearly and very gently at a distance of at least 5 mm and not to skeletonize it in order to avoid any injuries (→ p. 51, III-2)!

Follow the pathway of the nerve passing beneath the thyroid gland at its landmark, the so-called Zuckerkandle tubercle, up to its entry into the larynx.

Insert the caudal Langenbeck retractor again at the cranial margin of the incision. Then divide the distal branches of the inferior thyroid artery above a Mosquito hemostat step by step with Harmonic FOCUS® shears, close to the thyroid gland in order to protect the parathyroid vascular supply. Be aware of the recurrent laryngeal nerve during division of the artery to avoid any injuries.

> In case of a large diameter (> 5 mm) of the inferior thyroid artery, or if the artery runs too close to the recurrent laryngeal nerve, clip or ligate and divide the artery with curved scissors close to the thyroid gland (→ p. 51, III-1)!

> While dividing the inferior thyroid artery, pay attention to the recurrent laryngeal nerve in order to avoid any injuries (→ p. 51, III-2)!

Identifying and dissecting the recurrent laryngeal nerve

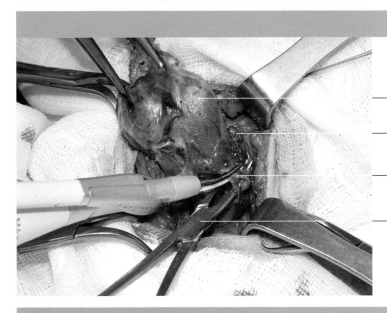

Zuckerkandle tubercle

Superior parathyroid gland

Thyroid lobe

Recurrent laryngeal nerve

Dividing the inferior thyroid artery

Thyroid lobe

Superior parathyroid gland

Inferior thyroid artery

Mosquito hemostat

Dividing the inferior thyroid artery

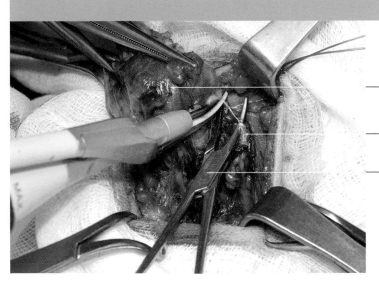

Thyroid lobe

Inferior thyroid artery

Mosquito hemostat

Nodal point 7   **Dissecting the inferior pole and dividing the inferior thyroid vein**

Incising the skin and the superficial cervical fascia

Exposing the thyroid

Preparing the thyroid and dividing the middle thyroid vein

Exposing the superior pole and dividing the superior thyroid vessels

Identifying the parathyroid glands

Identifying the recurrent laryngeal nerve and dividing the inferior thyroid artery

Dissecting the inferior pole and dividing the inferior thyroid vein

Mobilizing the thyroid lobe

Finishing the operation

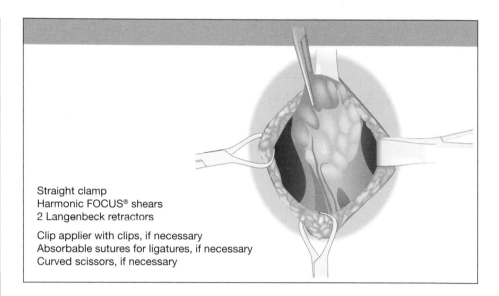

Straight clamp
Harmonic FOCUS® shears
2 Langenbeck retractors

Clip applier with clips, if necessary
Absorbable sutures for ligatures, if necessary
Curved scissors, if necessary

Retract the thyroid lobe cranially and to the opposite side with a straight clamp in order to expose the inferior pole. During dissection look for an accessory arteria thyroidea ima (Neubauer's artery), which in rare cases spreads from caudal into the inferior pole.

> Pay attention not to injure an existing accessory arteria thyroidea ima in order to avoid bleeding (→ p. 51, III-1)!

Separate the inferior pole and the inferior thyroid vein with Harmonic FOCUS® shears. Then seal the inferior thyroid vein with Harmonic FOCUS® shears.

> If the diameter of the inferior thyroid vein is too large (> 5 mm), it is mandatory to clip or ligate the vein with absorbable suture and to divide it with curved scissors (→ p. 51, III-1)!

Inferior pole

Inferior thyroid vein

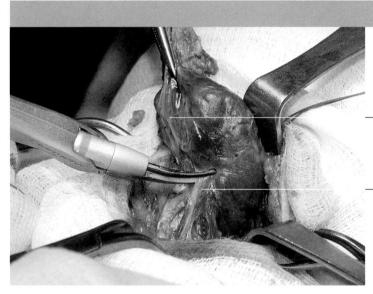

Inferior pole

Inferior thyroid vein

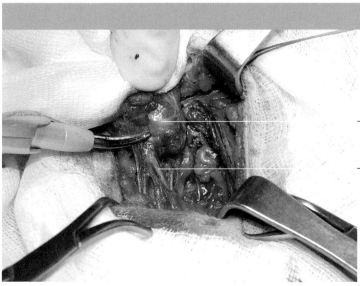

Thyroid lobe

Inferior thyroid vein

Nodal point 8   **Mobilizing the thyroid lobe**

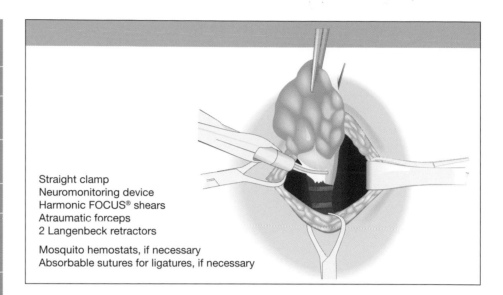

Straight clamp
Neuromonitoring device
Harmonic FOCUS® shears
Atraumatic forceps
2 Langenbeck retractors

Mosquito hemostats, if necessary
Absorbable sutures for ligatures, if necessary

Prior to the next step identify the recurrent laryngeal nerve and assess its functional integrity by using neuromonitoring. Follow the nerve until its entry under the cricothyroid muscle.

Release the thyroid lobe and the isthmus from the trachea by dissecting the posterior suspensory (Berry's) ligament with Harmonic FOCUS® shears without harming the trachea. Seal small blood vessels, running from the trachea to the thyroid gland with Harmonic FOCUS® shears.

> Be careful not to injure the trachea and to seal the small vessels in between the trachea and the thyroid gland in order to avoid any bleeding (→ p. 51, III-1; p. 52, III-5)!

Prepare the recurrent laryngeal nerve under vision systematically and very carefully free it from the thyroid lobe through the ligament of Berry with Harmonic FOCUS® shears. If the dissecting distance to the recurrent laryngeal nerve is less than 5 mm, release the thyroid lobe extremely carefully using Mosquito hemostats and ligatures.

> It is mandatory to separate the recurrent laryngeal nerve very cautiously from the thyroid lobe in order to avoid any injuries (→ p. 51, III-2)!

In case of a large struma, divide the isthmus with Harmonic FOCUS® shears.

After freeing the thyroid lobe, reposition the cranial Langenbeck retractor to the right lateral side of the incision in order to achieve a better view of the operative situs. Then check for bleeding and visualize the recurrent laryngeal nerve again.

For total struma resection, continue by preparing the contralateral side, starting again with nodal point 3.

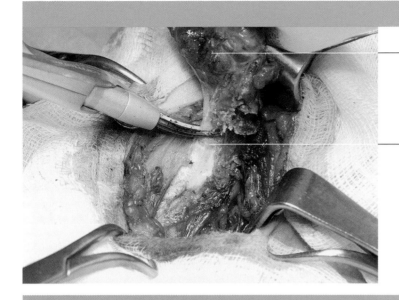

Thyroid lobe

Berry's ligament

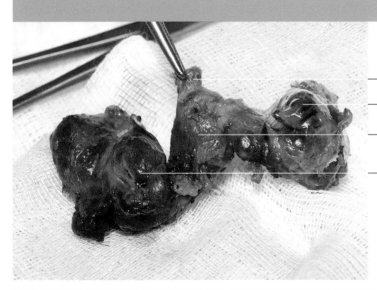

Pyramidal lobe

Left thyroid lobe

Isthmus

Right thyroid lobe

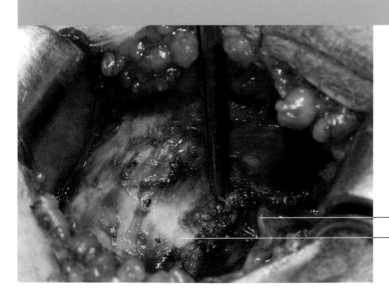

Recurrent laryngeal nerve

Trachea

Nodal point 9   Finishing the operation

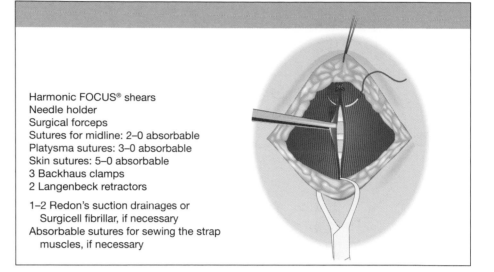

Harmonic FOCUS® shears
Needle holder
Surgical forceps
Sutures for midline: 2–0 absorbable
Platysma sutures: 3–0 absorbable
Skin sutures: 5–0 absorbable
3 Backhaus clamps
2 Langenbeck retractors

1–2 Redon's suction drainages or Surgicell fibrillar, if necessary
Absorbable sutures for sewing the strap muscles, if necessary

Re-check the operative situs for bleeding. Ask the anesthetist for a PEEP-ventilation (Valsalva's maneuver) in order to create overpressure in the thorax and thus to increase the filling of the blood vessels. Stop any visible bleeding with Harmonic FOCUS® shears.

> Make sure to stop any bleeding in the operative field in order to avoid post-operative bleeding (→ p. 51, III-1)!

Remove the two Langenbeck retractors and the two Backhaus clamps on both sides of the incision. Then reverse the hyperextension of the neck.

After removal of a large struma or in case of a large residual cavity in the neck, insert one or – if indicated – two Redon's suction drainages or Surgicell fibrillar.

If the strap muscles have been divided, sew them with absorbable suture. Adapt the strap muscles continuously with an absorbable thread to close the midline. Leave a window open in the inferior part of the midline in order to avoid pressure on the airways in case of postoperative bleeding into the thyroid bed.

> Take care to leave a window open in the inferior part of the midline in order to avoid high airway pressure in case of postoperative bleeding (→ p. 51, III-1)!

Remove the third Backhaus clamp and the retaining suture. Then suture the platysma and close the skin by a subcuticular suture with absorbable material. To achieve a good cosmetic result take care to sew the platysma separated from the skin.

> Be careful to sew the platysma separated from the skin in order to achieve a good cosmetic result!

Following disinfection, cover the wounds finally with sterile dressings.

> Postoperatively, it is mandatory to determine the calcium blood level and to test the function of the patient's vocal cords (→ p. 51, III-2; p. 52, III-6)!

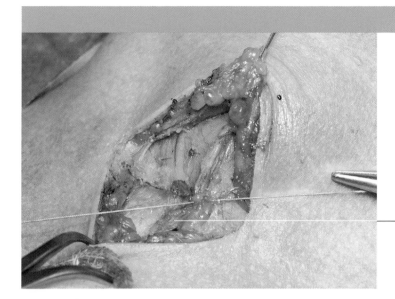

Strap muscles

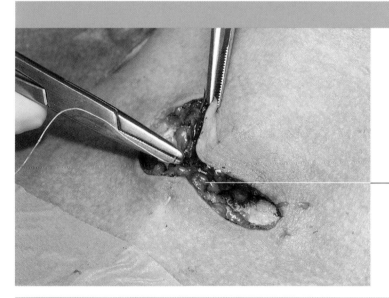

Subcutaneous fat and platysma

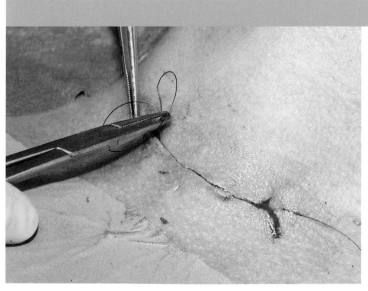

Management of difficult situations, complications and mistakes

In principle, to prevent any bleeding, pay attention to the anatomical details and perform an accurate intraoperative hemostasis!

a) Intraoperative bleeding

Coagulate the bleeding vessel with Harmonic FOCUS® shears or an electrocauter. If this does not terminate the bleeding, perform a ligature with absorbable suture.

b) Postoperative bleeding

Postoperative symptoms such as pain, increased diameter of neck with tension, increased blood drainage, respiratory distress and dysphagia are a distinct sign of postoperative bleeding.

In case of postoperative bleeding, the wound must be reopened immediately and the hematoma must be evacuated without any delay!

In the emergency of significant respiratory distress, an endotracheal intubation should be performed immediately!

The recurrent laryngeal nerve can be injured through stretching, cutting, clamping, thermal injury or compression (due to edema or hematoma).

If an injured recurrent laryngeal nerve is detected intraoperatively, suture the nerve using microsurgical techniques.

a) Unilateral injury

In case of postoperative hoarseness and/or voice alteration, the patient should receive vocal therapy from a speech-language pathologist.

If the injury is declared permanent, the injection of silicone or microsurgery of the cords in specialized otorhinolaryngologist units could be a therapeutic option.

b) Bilateral injury

In case of serious postoperative dyspnea with stridor, perform a laryngoscopy and reintubate the patient at once. Begin intravenous treatment with corticosteroids, antiphlogistics and calcium.

In case of a persisting respiratory obstruction, perform a permanent tracheotomy or a transverse laser cordotomy to open a window on the cords. Should the occasion arise, conduct a lateralization of the vocal cords to avoid a permanent tracheotomy.

In case of any neural injuries ask for the advice of an otorhinolaryngologist postoperatively!

3 Injury to the external branch of the superior laryngeal nerve

Injury to the external branch of the superior laryngeal nerve can occur during the preparation of the superior pole. Such an injury leads to an inability to perform higher-piched vocal sounds.

In case of postoperative voice alteration, the patient should receive vocal therapy from a speech-language pathologist.

In case of any neural injuries ask for the advice of an otorhinolaryngologist postoperatively!

4 Injury of the pericarotid plexus

Injury to the cervical sympathetic trunk running next to the carotid sheath can occur during preparation of the lateral part of the thyroid lobe in deeper tissue layers. Such an injury can cause Horner's syndrome, which is characterized by facial dryness, a constricted pupil and a drooping eyelid.

As there is no possibility to treat a Horner's syndrome, enlight the patient preoperatively about this rarely complication, particularly if you perform a lateral lymphadenectomy for cancer.

5 Injury to the trachea

Injury to the trachea can occur while the thyroid gland is being released from the trachea.

In case of a perforation, suture the trachea immediately after resection of the damaged part of the trachea. Cover the suture with vital tissue, for example a muscle flap, if necessary.

Following injury to the trachea, postoperative bronchoscopy is mandatory!

6 Injury to the parathyroid glands

If the parathyroid glands or their vascular supply have been injured during their separation from the posterior capsule of the thyroid, implant them into the sternocleidomastoid muscle or another appropriate muscle at the time of thyroidectomy to prevent postoperative hypoparathyroidism and hypocalcemia.

Treat postoperatively diagnosed hypoparathyroidism and hypocalcemia with calcium and vitamin D.

Anatomical variations

The relationship between the recurrent laryngeal nerve and the inferior thyroid artery is very variable, particularly on the right side.

The recurrent laryngeal nerve passes the inferior thyroid artery dorsally.

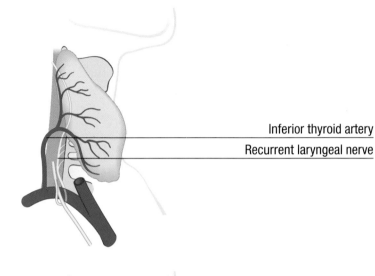

Inferior thyroid artery

Recurrent laryngeal nerve

The recurrent laryngeal nerve runs superficial to the inferior thyroid artery.

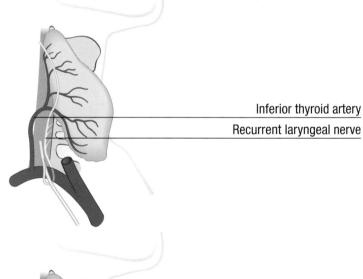

Inferior thyroid artery

Recurrent laryngeal nerve

The recurrent laryngeal nerve passes between the branches of the inferior thyroid artery.

Inferior thyroid artery

Recurrent laryngeal nerve

Neural variations

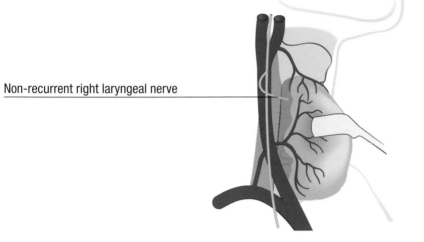

The non-recurrent right laryngeal nerve runs directly to the larynx.

Non-recurrent right laryngeal nerve

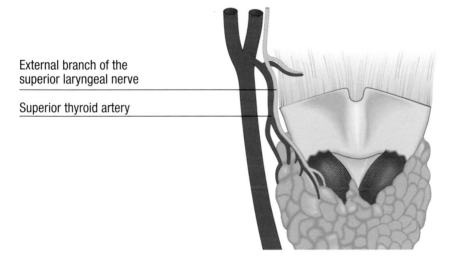

The external branch of the superior laryngeal nerve runs medial to or around the superior thyroid artery.

External branch of the superior laryngeal nerve

Superior thyroid artery

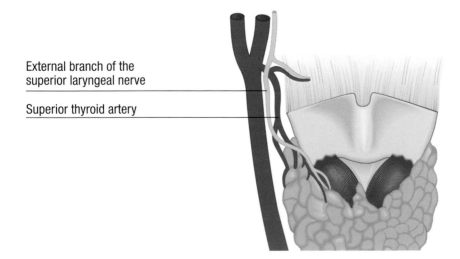

The external branch of the superior laryngeal nerve crosses the superior thyroid artery at the height of the superior thyroid pole.

External branch of the superior laryngeal nerve

Superior thyroid artery

An accessory arteria thyroidea ima (Neubauer's artery) originates from the brachiocephalic trunk, the right carotid artery, directly from the aortic arch, the internal thoracic artery or from a mediastinal artery. The arteria ima runs ventral to the trachea cranially to the thyroid gland and spreads into the inferior pole.

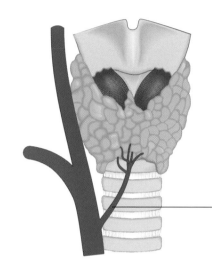

Accessory arteria thyroidea ima

The superior and inferior parathyroid glands are supplied by a single branch of the inferior thyroid artery.

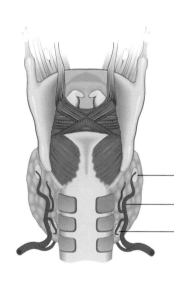

Superior parathyroid gland

Inferior thyroid artery

Inferior parathyroid gland

The superior and inferior parathyroid glands are supplied by multiple branches of the inferior thyroid artery.

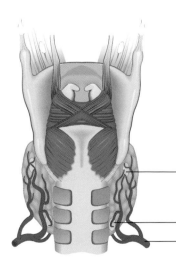

Superior parathyroid gland

Inferior parathyroid gland

Inferior thyroid artery

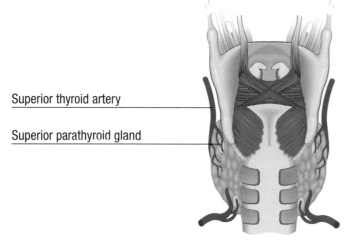

Superior thyroid artery

Superior parathyroid gland

The superior parathyroid gland is supplied by the superior thyroid artery.

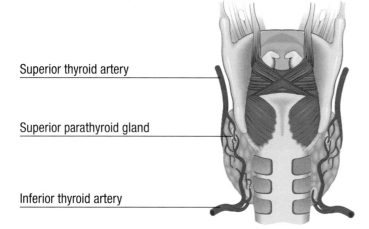

Superior thyroid artery

Superior parathyroid gland

Inferior thyroid artery

The superior parathyroid gland receives its blood from the inferior and superior thyroid artery.

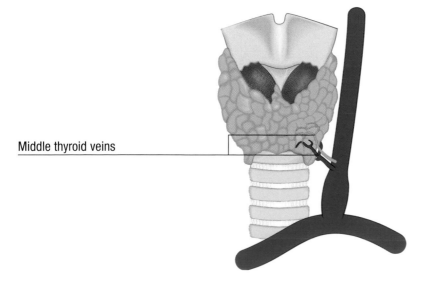

Middle thyroid veins

Middle thyroid veins vary in number.

There are variable positions of ectopic parathyroid glands, particularly of the inferior parathyroid gland. The figure shows the sections in which the superior and inferior ectopic parathyroid glands can be found.

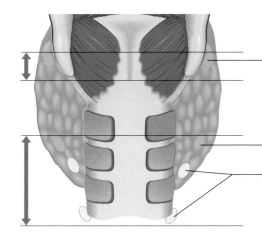

Superior parathyroid gland

Inferior parathyroid gland

Ectopic inferior parathyroid glands

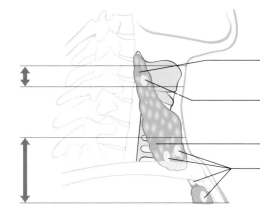

Superior parathyroid gland

Ectopic superior parathyroid gland

Inferior parathyroid gland

Ectopic inferior parathyroid glands

Sample operation note

59

Bibliography

List of key words

Sample operation note

Date:	Operating surgeon:
Patient's name:	Assistant:
Operation diagnosis: Multinodular goiter	Instrument nurse:
Operation: Thyroidectomy with Harmonic FOCUS® shears	Anesthetist:

A curvilinear collar-type skin incision is made 2 cm above the sternal notch. Upper and lower skin flaps are created; a retaining suture is positioned. The skin flaps are dissected away from the strap muscles in an avascular plane with preservation of the anterior jugular veins. Strap muscles are split in the midline. Small crossing vessels are treated using Harmonic FOCUS® shears, and strap muscles on both sides are dissected from the thyroid capsule.

The left lobe is dissected first. The forefront of the thyroid lobe is prepared progressively toward lateral, up to the carotid sheath. The lobe is gently pulled out from the wound. The middle thyroid vein is coagulated and cut with Harmonic FOCUS® shears. The superior thyroid pole is dissected from the cricothyroid muscle. After the external branch of the superior laryngeal nerve has been exposed, using neuromonitoring (if present), a window is opened medially between the cricothyroid muscle and the superior pole. The superior thyroid vessels are coagulated and cut with Harmonic FOCUS® shears. The lobe is rotated medially and mobilized anteriorly.

The parathyroid glands are identified and dissected from the thyroid capsule. The recurrent laryngeal nerve is identified and dissected, using neuromonitoring, until its entrance into the larynx. Small terminal branches of the inferior thyroid artery are cut with Harmonic FOCUS® shears, preserving the parathyroid vascularization.

The inferior thyroid pole is separated and the inferior thyroid vein is coagulated and cut with Harmonic FOCUS® shears. The left lobe is dissected away from the trachea under constant control of the recurrent laryngeal nerve using neuromonitoring. Finally, Berry's ligament is cut and the lobectomy is completed.

The right lobe is then prepared and resected using the same technique as described for the left lobe.

After the thyroidectomy is completed, the operative situs is checked for bleeding. Visible bleeding is arrested with Harmonic FOCUS® shears. The strap muscles are adapted with absorbable sutures, leaving the lower part of the midline wide open. The platysma is approximated with absorbable stitches and the skin is closed with an intradermal running suture.

Carpenter W.B. (1874). *Principles of Mental Physiology: With their Applications to the Training and Discipline of the Mind and the Study of its Comorbid Conditions.* London: Henry S. King & Co.

Cordón C., Fajardo R., Ramírez J. & Herrera F. (2005). A randomized, prospective, parallel group study comparing the Harmonic Scalpel to electrocautery in the thyroidectomy. *Surgery,* 137: 337-341.

Defechereux T., Rinken F., Maweja E., Hamoir E. & Meurisse M. (2003). Evaluation of the ultrasonic dissector in thyroid surgery. A prospective randomised study. *Acta Chirurgica Belgica,* 103: 274-277.

Eberspächer H. (2001). *Mentales Training.* München: Copress.

Feltz D.L. & Landers D.M. (1983). The effects of mental practice on motor skill learning and performance: A meta-analysis. *Journal of Sport Psychology,* 5: 25-57.

Güler A.K., Immenroth M., Berg T., Bürger T. & Gawad K.A. (2006). Evaluation einer neu konzipierten Operationsfibel durch den Vergleich mit einer klassischen Operationslehre. *Posterpräsentation auf dem 123. Kongress der Deutschen Gesellschaft für Chirurgie vom 02.–05. Mai 2006 in Berlin.*

Immenroth M. (2003). *Mentales Training in der Medizin. Anwendung in der Chirurgie und Zahnmedizin.* Hamburg: Kovač.

Immenroth M., Bürger T., Brenner J., Kemmler R., Nagelschmidt R., Eberspächer H. & Troidl H. (2005). Mentales Training in der Chirurgie. *Der Chirurg* BDC, 44(1): 21-25.

Immenroth M., Bürger T., Brenner J., Nagelschmidt R., Eberspächer H. & Troidl H. (2007). Mental Training in surgical education: A randomized controlled trial. *Annals of Surgery,* 245: 385-391.

Immenroth M., Eberspächer H. & Hermann H.D. (2008). Training kognitiver Fertigkeiten. In J. Beckmann & M. Kellmann (Hrsg.), *Enzyklopädie der Psychologie (D, V, 2) Anwendungen der Sportpsychologie* (119-176). Göttingen: Hogrefe.

Immenroth M., Eberspächer H., Nagelschmidt M., Troidl H., Bürger T., Brenner J., Berg T., Müller M. & Kemmler R. (2005). Mentales Training in der Chirurgie – Sicherheit durch ein besseres Training. Design und erste Ergebnisse einer Studie. *MIC,* 14: 69-74.

Lotze R.H. (1852). *Medicinische Psychologie und Physiologie der Seele.* Leipzig: Weidmann'sche Buchhandlung.

Bibliography

Miccoli P., Berti P., Dionigi G.L., D'Agostino J., Orlandini C. & Donatini G. (2006). Randomized controlled trial of Harmonic Scalpel use during thyroidectomy. *Archives of Otolaryngology-Head & Neck Surgery,* 132: 1069-1073.

Middelanis I., Liehn M., Steinmüller L. & Döhler J.R. (2003). *OP-Handbuch.* Berlin, Heidelberg, New York: Springer Verlag.

Miller G.A. (1956). The magical number seven plus or minus two: Some limits on our capacity for processing information. *Psychological Review,* 63: 81-97.

Netter F.H. (2000). *Atlas der Anatomie des Menschen.* Stuttgart, New York: Georg Thieme Verlag.

Oertli D. & Udelsman R. (2007). *Surgery of the thyroid and the parathyroid glands.* Berlin, Heidelberg, New York: Springer Verlag.

Rehner M. & Oestern H.J. (1997). *Chirurgische Facharztweiterbildung,* Band 1. Stuttgart, New York: Georg Thieme Verlag.

Voutilainen P.E. & Haglund C.H. (2000). Ultrasonically activated shears in thyroidectomies. A randomized trial. *Annals of Surgery,* 231: 322-328.

Titles available

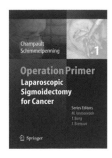 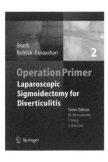 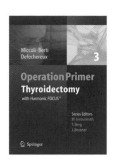

Volume 1: Laparoscopic Sigmoidectomy for Cancer	ISBN 978-3-540-78453-1
Volume 2: Laparoscopic Sigmoidectomy for Diverticulitis	ISBN 978-3-540-78451-7
Volume 3: Thyroidectomy with Harmonic FOCUS®	ISBN 978-3-540-85163-9

Titles in preparation

Laparoscopic total Mesorectal Excision (TME) for Cancer

Laparoscopic Cholecystectomy

Clipless Laparoscopic Cholecystectomy with Harmonic® shears

Laparoscopic Gastric Banding with the Swedish Adjustable Gastric Band (SAGB VC)

Stapled Transanal Rectal Resection (STARR) with Contour® Transtar™ Curved Cutter Stapler Procedure Set

Open Rectal Resection

Notes

Notes